HEALTHY HABITS HAPPY KIDS

Navigating the Challenges of Childhood Obesity

JULIAN TIM

TABLE OF CONTENTS

INTRODUCTION

In a world where the rhythms of modern life often clash with the essence of childhood, Julian Tim invites you on a transformative journey within the pages of "Healthy Habits, Happy Kids: Navigating the Challenges of Childhood Obesity." As an Amazon publisher and fervent advocate for children's well-being, Tim intricately weaves together expertise and empathy to address one of the most pressing issues of our time – childhood obesity.

In this insightful exploration, you'll embark on a quest to cultivate a foundation of health that will resonate throughout a lifetime. The pages of this book serve as a compass, guiding parents and caregivers through the labyrinth of nutritional choices, lifestyle adjustments, and mindful parenting. Tim, with a unique blend of medical knowledge and storytelling finesse, unveils the complexities of childhood obesity while offering practical solutions with a compassionate touch.

"Healthy Habits, Happy Kids" is not merely a guide; it's a narrative of empowerment. Each chapter unfolds like a conversation with a trusted friend, providing a roadmap for instilling habits that promote vitality, resilience, and joy in our children. From navigating the grocery store aisles to fostering positive body image, this book is a comprehensive toolkit designed to equip families with the tools they need to navigate the challenges of raising healthy, happy kids.

As you delve into these pages, you'll discover more than advice – you'll find a source of inspiration and a call to action. Join Julian Tim on this transformative expedition, where the pursuit of health becomes a celebration of the unique vibrancy within each child. "Healthy Habits, Happy Kids" is not just a book; it's a beacon of hope, a manual for building a future where our children thrive physically, emotionally, and holistically.

CHAPTER 1

UNDERSTANDING CHILDHOOD OBESITY

Childhood obesity refers to a medical condition characterized by excessive body fat accumulation in children and adolescents. This condition has become a significant public health concern globally due to its prevalence and associated health risks. The primary factor contributing to childhood obesity is an imbalance between calorie intake and energy expenditure. Factors such as unhealthy eating habits, sedentary lifestyles, and genetic predispositions can contribute to the development of obesity in children.

The consequences of childhood obesity extend beyond physical health, impacting psychological and social well-being. Children who experience obesity may face increased risks of developing various health issues, including type 2 diabetes, cardiovascular diseases, and orthopedic problems. Additionally, the psychological impact can manifest as low self-esteem, depression, and social isolation, as children may face bullying or stigma related to their weight.

Preventing childhood obesity involves a multi-faceted approach, including promoting healthy eating habits, encouraging physical activity, and addressing environmental factors that contribute to an obesogenic environment. Interventions at the individual, family, community, and policy levels are crucial to combating this issue. Schools, healthcare providers, and parents play pivotal roles in educating children about nutrition, fostering physical activity, and creating supportive environments that promote a healthy lifestyle.

It is essential to recognize that childhood obesity is a complex issue influenced by a combination of genetic, behavioral, and environmental factors. Tackling this problem requires collaborative efforts from various stakeholders to implement effective strategies that promote overall health and well-being in children.

Impacts of Childhood Obesity

Childhood obesity has profound and far-reaching impacts on various aspects of a child's life. One of the most immediate consequences is the negative effect on physical health. Children with obesity are at a higher risk of developing a range of health issues, including type 2 diabetes, cardiovascular diseases, and respiratory problems. These health complications can persist into adulthood, potentially shortening the individual's lifespan and contributing to an increased burden on healthcare systems.

Beyond the physical implications, childhood obesity significantly affects mental and emotional well-being. Children who experience obesity often face social stigma, bullying, and discrimination, leading to psychological distress and a higher likelihood of developing mental health issues such as depression and anxiety. The negative impact on self-esteem can be long-lasting, influencing various aspects of a child's social interactions, academic performance, and overall quality of life.

Educational outcomes are also affected by childhood obesity. Research indicates that obese children may experience challenges in academic achievement, cognitive functioning, and classroom behavior. This can create a cycle of disadvantage, as the psychological and social consequences of obesity may hinder a child's ability to engage effectively in educational settings, limiting their future opportunities and success.

The economic impact of childhood obesity is substantial, affecting not only healthcare costs but also productivity and societal well-being. The increased prevalence of obesity-related health conditions in children places a significant financial burden on healthcare systems, diverting resources that could be allocated elsewhere. Additionally, the long-term consequences of childhood obesity, such as reduced productivity and increased absenteeism, contribute to economic challenges on a broader scale.

Family dynamics are also influenced by childhood obesity. Parents and caregivers may experience emotional distress and feelings of guilt, and family relationships can be strained as efforts to address the child's weight become a central focus. Furthermore, the entire family may be susceptible to adopting unhealthy lifestyle habits, perpetuating a cycle of obesity across generations.

In summary, childhood obesity has a multifaceted impact on physical health, mental well-being, educational outcomes, economic stability, and family dynamics. Addressing this issue requires comprehensive strategies that encompass healthcare, education, community support, and policy interventions to create environments that promote healthy living and prevent the long-term consequences of obesity in children.

Setting the Stage for Lasting Change

In the realm of childhood obesity, establishing lasting change is not only about addressing the symptoms but delving into the root causes and building a foundation for sustainable habits. This section of the book emphasizes the importance of creating an environment conducive to positive health outcomes for children. It recognizes that lasting change involves a comprehensive approach that extends beyond individual behaviors to encompass familial, societal, and environmental factors.

The chapter begins by acknowledging the complexities surrounding childhood obesity, emphasizing that a nuanced understanding is crucial for effective intervention. It delves into the role of parents, caregivers, and educators in shaping a child's lifestyle and cultivating habits that promote well-being. By providing practical guidance and evidence-based strategies, the book empowers readers to initiate meaningful changes in daily routines, dietary choices, and physical activities, laying the groundwork for a healthier lifestyle.

Also, the significance of community engagement and support networks. Recognizing that healthy habits are reinforced by social influences, the book encourages readers to become advocates for change within their communities. It discusses how schools, healthcare systems, and local organizations can play integral roles in fostering an environment that prioritizes the well-being of children and addresses the broader societal factors contributing to childhood obesity.

Moreover, this section emphasizes the need for policy interventions to create a systemic impact. By advocating for policies that promote healthier food options, increased physical activity in schools, and improved urban planning to facilitate active lifestyles, the book guides readers towards becoming agents of change on a larger scale. It underscores the interconnectedness of individual choices and the broader societal context, reinforcing the idea that lasting change requires a collective effort.

Moreover, it sets the tone for proactive and enduring solutions to childhood obesity. It empowers readers with knowledge, tools, and a holistic perspective, encouraging them to become catalysts for change within their families, communities, and society at large. Through this section, the book positions itself as a guide not only for navigating the challenges of childhood obesity but for instigating transformative and enduring shifts in the way we approach children's health.

CHAPTER 2

THE FOUNDATION:BUILDING A NUTRIENT-RICH ENVIRONMENT

Childhood obesity is a pressing concern, demanding a comprehensive foundation for a nutrient-rich environment. Beyond dietary considerations, this foundation encompasses various aspects of a child's life contributing to overall well-being.

Implementing educational programs in schools and communities empowers children and parents with essential nutritional knowledge. These initiatives cover balanced diets, portion control, and the importance of diverse food groups.

Encouraging regular physical activity is pivotal. Schools can incorporate engaging exercise routines into the curriculum, fostering a love for movement. Community spaces can be designed to promote active play.

Ensuring accessible, nutritious meals for all children, irrespective of socio-economic backgrounds, involves collaborations with local farmers, subsidizing healthy options, or implementing school meal programs prioritizing nutrient-rich ingredients.

Active parental involvement is crucial. Workshops, support groups, and informative sessions provide parents with tools and knowledge for creating a healthy home environment.

Equipping children with basic culinary skills instills responsibility and a connection between food and nutrition. This includes teaching them how to prepare simple, nutritious meals.

Promoting mindful eating habits helps prevent overeating. Encouraging children to savor each bite and pay attention to hunger and fullness cues establishes a healthy relationship with food.

Addressing the impact of technology on nutrition is essential. Educating parents and children about the potential pitfalls of excessive screen time helps combat sedentary behavior and unhealthy eating habits.

Community gardens offer a hands-on approach. Children actively participating in growing fruits and vegetables fosters a connection to fresh produce and a sense of pride.

Regular health check-ups are vital for monitoring growth, development, and nutritional status in children. Early identification of health issues allows for timely intervention.

Recognizing the psychological aspects of childhood obesity is crucial. Implementing programs that address body image, self-esteem, and stress management creates a holistic approach to well-being.

Establishing policy advocacy is necessary. Collaborating with policymakers to implement regulations prioritizing nutrition in schools, public spaces, and children-targeted food advertising supports a nutrient-rich environment

Nutritional Essentials for Growing Bodies

Proper nutrition plays a pivotal role in the healthy development of growing bodies. In the formative years of childhood, it is crucial to understand the nutritional essentials that contribute to overall well-being. The foundation of a healthy diet for growing bodies lies in a balance of macronutrients—carbohydrates, proteins, and fats. Carbohydrates serve as the primary energy source, while proteins are vital for muscle development and repair. Healthy fats, such as those found in avocados and nuts, are essential for brain development and overall cellular function.

Micronutrients, including vitamins and minerals, are equally vital for growing bodies. These nutrients contribute to various physiological processes, such as bone development, immune function, and metabolic regulation. A diverse and colorful diet, encompassing a range of fruits and vegetables, ensures a broad spectrum of essential vitamins and minerals. For example, vitamin D is crucial for calcium absorption and bone health, while iron supports oxygen transport in the blood.

As children transition through different stages of growth, their nutritional needs evolve. Infants, for instance, rely on breast milk or formula as their primary source of nutrition, providing essential nutrients for rapid development. Introducing a variety of solid foods as they approach six months of age helps expose them to different tastes and textures, fostering healthy eating habits from an early age. In adolescence, with the onset of puberty and growth spurts, nutritional requirements increase, emphasizing the importance of balanced meals and snacks.

Encouraging healthy eating habits is fundamental to instilling a positive relationship with food in growing children. Parents and caregivers can play a pivotal role by creating a supportive food environment. This includes offering a variety of nutrient-dense foods, involving children in meal planning and preparation, and establishing regular mealtimes. Modeling healthy eating behaviors and maintaining a positive attitude toward food can significantly influence a child's dietary choices and preferences.

Adequate hydration is often overlooked but is a critical component of proper nutrition for growing bodies. Water is essential for various bodily functions, including digestion, nutrient transport, and temperature regulation. Ensuring that children have access to water throughout the day and encouraging them to stay hydrated supports overall health and well-being.

Despite the importance of essential nutrients, it's essential to be mindful of portion sizes. Understanding age-appropriate serving sizes prevents overconsumption and helps maintain a healthy weight. Teaching children to listen to their body's hunger and fullness cues fosters a sense of intuitive eating, promoting a balanced relationship with food.

In the modern environment, where processed and convenience foods are prevalent, educating families about making informed nutritional choices is crucial. Reading food labels, identifying hidden sugars, and choosing whole, minimally processed foods contribute to a nutrient-rich diet. By empowering parents with the knowledge to make informed choices, the aim is to create a supportive nutritional environment that sets the stage for a lifetime of healthy habits.

Nutritional essentials for growing bodies encompass a well-balanced diet rich in macronutrients, micronutrients, and hydration. Cultivating healthy eating habits, understanding evolving nutritional needs through different developmental stages, and making informed choices contribute to the overall health and well-being of growing children. By focusing on these nutritional principles, we lay the groundwork for a healthier future generation.

Creating Balanced and Delicious Meals

Balancing nutrition and taste is key to fostering healthy eating habits, especially in the context of growing bodies. Start by incorporating a variety of colorful fruits and vegetables into meals. These vibrant foods provide an array of vitamins, minerals, and antioxidants essential for overall health. Aim to include a mix of leafy greens, bright berries, and diverse vegetables to create visually appealing and nutritionally rich dishes.

Incorporating lean proteins into meals is crucial for growth and muscle development. Opt for sources like poultry, fish, tofu, legumes, and nuts to ensure a balance of essential amino acids. Experiment with different cooking methods, such as grilling, baking, or sautéing, to add variety and enhance flavors. Including protein-rich ingredients not only contributes to nutritional needs but also helps create satisfying and delicious meals.

Whole grains are a fundamental component of a balanced diet. Swap refined grains for whole grains like quinoa, brown rice, or whole wheat to increase fiber content and provide sustained energy. These grains add texture and depth to meals while promoting digestive health. Create delightful grain bowls, incorporating a mix of colorful vegetables, proteins, and flavorful sauces for a well-rounded and tasty dining experience.

Balanced meals should include healthy fats, such as those found in avocados, olive oil, and nuts. These fats are essential for brain development, nutrient absorption, and overall cellular function. Experiment with incorporating these fats into dressings, spreads, or as toppings to enhance both the nutritional profile and taste of your meals.

Herbs and spices are invaluable for elevating the flavor of meals without relying on excessive salt or sugar. Experiment with a variety of herbs like basil, cilantro, and mint, along with spices such as cumin, paprika, and turmeric. These additions not only enhance the taste but also contribute antioxidants and anti-inflammatory properties, enhancing the overall health benefits of the meal.

When planning meals, consider the importance of proper portion sizes. Avoid the temptation to supersize meals, as this can lead to overconsumption of calories. Use smaller plates to create the illusion of a fuller plate while maintaining appropriate portion control. This strategy promotes mindful eating, allowing individuals to savor each bite and recognize their body's hunger and fullness cues.

Involving children in the meal preparation process can foster a positive relationship with food. Encourage them to choose ingredients, assist in cooking, and explore various flavors. This hands-on approach not only makes mealtime an interactive and enjoyable experience but also instills a sense of responsibility and appreciation for healthy food choices.

Lastly, maintain flexibility and creativity in your approach to cooking. Experiment with new recipes, try diverse cuisines, and adapt meals based on seasonal produce. By keeping meals interesting and flavorful, you can ensure that healthy eating remains an exciting and sustainable part of your lifestyle. In creating balanced and delicious meals, you're not only nourishing your body but also cultivating a love for nutritious foods that lasts a lifetime.

CHAPTER 3

BEYOND THE PLATE: HOLISTIC LIFESTYLE PRACTICES

Beyond the plate, holistic lifestyle practices encompass a range of habits that contribute to overall well-being. One fundamental aspect is getting enough quality sleep. Establish a consistent sleep routine, create a relaxing bedtime environment, and aim for 7-9 hours of sleep each night. Quality sleep is crucial for physical and mental health.

Incorporate regular physical activity into your routine. Find activities you enjoy, whether it's walking, yoga, or dancing, and make them a consistent part of your schedule. Exercise not only improves physical health but also boosts mood and enhances overall vitality.

Practice mindfulness and stress reduction techniques. This can include meditation, deep breathing exercises, or simply taking moments throughout the day to be present. Mindfulness contributes to mental clarity, reduced stress levels, and a greater sense of calm.

Stay hydrated by drinking an adequate amount of water throughout the day. Proper hydration supports various bodily functions, including digestion, circulation, and temperature regulation. Consider carrying a reusable water bottle to encourage consistent water intake.

Cultivate meaningful connections with others. Social relationships play a vital role in holistic well-being. Nurture your friendships, spend quality time with loved ones, and engage in activities that foster a sense of community and belonging.

Prioritize mental health by seeking professional support when needed. A therapist or counselor can provide valuable tools and strategies for managing stress, anxiety, or other mental health challenges. Taking care of your mental well-being is an integral part of a holistic lifestyle.

Embrace a balanced approach to technology use. Set boundaries on screen time, especially before bedtime, to promote better sleep. Consider incorporating tech-free periods during the day to foster real-world connections and reduce digital-related stress.

Create a positive and inspiring living environment. Declutter spaces, personalize your surroundings, and incorporate elements that bring joy and relaxation. A harmonious home environment positively influences overall well-being.

Practice gratitude by regularly reflecting on the positive aspects of your life. Keep a gratitude journal or simply take a moment each day to acknowledge and appreciate the things you are thankful for. Cultivating gratitude fosters a positive mindset.

Explore holistic nutrition by focusing on whole, nutrient-dense foods. Incorporate a variety of fruits, vegetables, lean proteins, and whole grains into your meals. Pay attention to how different foods make you feel and prioritize those that contribute to sustained energy and well-being.

Engage in continuous learning and personal growth. Challenge yourself with new experiences, hobbies, or educational pursuits. Lifelong learning fosters a sense of accomplishment, stimulates the mind, and contributes to a fulfilling life.

Practice self-compassion and self-care. Be kind to yourself, acknowledge your achievements, and prioritize activities that bring you joy and relaxation. Taking time for self-care is essential for maintaining balance and preventing burnout.

By incorporating these holistic lifestyle practices beyond the plate, you can create a well-rounded approach to health and well-being that extends to various aspects of your life. These habits contribute to a more vibrant, fulfilling, and balanced lifestyle.

The Role of Physical Activity in Curbing Childhood Obesity in a Sedentary World

In the battle against childhood obesity within our increasingly sedentary world, understanding and emphasizing the role of physical activity is paramount. Begin by recognizing the importance of setting a positive example. Parents, caregivers, and educators play influential roles in shaping children's behaviors. By incorporating regular physical activity into their own routines and making it a family priority, adults can instill the value of movement from an early age.

Introduce play as a form of exercise. Engaging in active play is not only enjoyable for children but also an effective way to ensure they get the recommended amount of physical activity. Encourage activities that involve running, jumping, climbing, and playing games that enhance coordination and motor skills. Making physical activity fun fosters a positive association, making children more likely to embrace an active lifestyle.

Limit screen time and encourage outdoor play. In a world dominated by screens, it's crucial to set guidelines on recreational screen use. Encourage outdoor activities that stimulate physical movement, such as biking, playing sports, or simply running around in the backyard. Creating a balance between screen time and outdoor play helps mitigate sedentary behavior and contributes to overall health.

Incorporate physical activity into daily routines. Look for opportunities to infuse movement into everyday activities. Walking or biking to school, engaging in active chores, and incorporating short bursts of physical activity during study breaks are effective ways to counteract sedentary behavior. These small, consistent efforts add up over time, contributing to a healthier lifestyle.

Promote organized sports and physical education. Organized sports not only provide a structured way for children to engage in physical activity but also foster teamwork, discipline, and skill development. Advocate for the inclusion of quality physical education programs in schools, ensuring that children receive adequate opportunities for movement and exercise during the school day.

Encourage active commuting. Where feasible, promote walking or biking to school as an alternative to passive transportation. This not only contributes to daily physical activity but also instills a sense of independence and environmental awareness. Work with communities to create safe routes for active commuting, fostering a culture that values movement.

Integrate technology with physical activity. Recognizing the prevalence of technology in children's lives, leverage it to promote movement. Explore interactive video games that require physical activity, use fitness apps designed for children, or incorporate virtual fitness challenges. This approach combines technology with physical activity, making it more engaging for tech-savvy youngsters.

Create a supportive environment. Schools, communities, and families should collaborate to create environments that encourage and facilitate physical activity. This may involve developing safe playgrounds, organizing community sports events, and advocating for policies that prioritize physical education and recreational spaces.

Emphasize the importance of diverse activities. Children have different interests and abilities, so it's crucial to offer a variety of physical activities. Whether it's dance, swimming, martial arts, or team sports, providing options ensures that children can find activities they enjoy, increasing the likelihood of sustained participation.

Monitor and celebrate progress. Keep track of children's physical activity levels and celebrate their achievements. Recognize improvements, whether in endurance, skills, or participation. Positive reinforcement and encouragement play a vital role in fostering a lifelong commitment to physical activity.

Combating childhood obesity in a sedentary world requires a multifaceted approach, with a central focus on the role of physical activity. By integrating movement into various aspects of children's lives and creating a supportive environment, we can significantly contribute to the prevention and reduction of childhood obesity, promoting a healthier and more active future generation.

Prioritizing Sleep and Stress Management

Childhood obesity has become a pressing public health concern, necessitating a comprehensive strategy that extends beyond dietary considerations. Prioritizing adequate sleep and effective stress management is emerging as a crucial component in addressing and preventing obesity in children.

Insufficient sleep has been consistently linked to an increased risk of childhood obesity. Research suggests that sleep deprivation disrupts the delicate hormonal balance responsible for appetite regulation, leading to heightened cravings for high-calorie foods and subsequent weight gain. Encouraging consistent sleep patterns in children is paramount to breaking this cycle.

In the modern digital age, excessive screen time has become a pervasive issue among children, contributing to both poor sleep quality and increased stress levels. Establishing limits on screen time and promoting outdoor activities not only addresses sedentary behavior but also positively impacts sleep, creating a healthier lifestyle overall.

Stress plays a significant role in the development of unhealthy eating habits and disrupted sleep patterns in children. Teaching stress management techniques, such as mindfulness and relaxation exercises, equips children with valuable tools to navigate life's challenges while mitigating the risk of obesity.

Consistency is key in promoting healthy sleep and stress management habits. Establishing regular routines provides children with stability, positively impacting their physical and mental well-being. Parental involvement is crucial in creating a supportive environment, fostering open communication, and ensuring that sleep is prioritized in the family routine.

Nutritional choices can influence both sleep quality and obesity risk. A well-balanced diet, rich in sleep-promoting nutrients like tryptophan and magnesium, can indirectly contribute to weight management. Educating children about the connection between nutrition, sleep, and overall health empowers them to make informed choices.

Regular physical activity is not only essential for weight management but also contributes to better sleep quality. Encouraging children to engage in age-appropriate exercises fosters a healthy lifestyle, addressing both physical and mental well-being.

Promoting good sleep hygiene practices is crucial. Educating children about the importance of a comfortable sleep environment, consistent bedtime routines, and minimizing external disruptions contributes to the development of healthy sleep habits.

Addressing environmental factors is equally important. Noise, light, and electronic devices can disrupt sleep patterns. Creating a conducive sleep environment involves minimizing these external disturbances, fostering an atmosphere conducive to restful sleep.

Collaborative efforts from schools, healthcare providers, and communities are essential in raising awareness about the interconnectedness of sleep, stress, and obesity. Implementing educational programs and providing resources empowers families to make informed choices and prioritize the well-being of their children.

prioritizing sleep and stress management is integral to a holistic approach in curbing childhood obesity. By addressing these fundamental aspects, we not only contribute to the immediate health of children but also lay the groundwork for healthier habits that can extend into adulthood, fostering a society that values overall well-being.

Twenty Healthy Sleeping Habits to Cultivate in Children

1. Consistent Bedtime Routine: Establish a regular bedtime routine to signal to the child that it's time to wind down and prepare for sleep.

2. Consistent Sleep Schedule: Maintain a consistent sleep schedule, even on weekends, to regulate the child's internal body clock.

3. Create a Comfortable Sleep Environment: Ensure the child's bedroom is conducive to sleep by maintaining a comfortable

temperature, minimizing noise, and using blackout curtains.

4. Limit Screen Time Before Bed: Reduce exposure to screens at least an hour before bedtime to minimize the impact of blue light on melatonin production.

5. Encourage Relaxing Activities: Prioritize calming activities before bedtime, such as reading a book, taking a warm bath, or practicing gentle stretching exercises.

6. Adequate Physical Activity: Ensure the child engages in age-appropriate

physical activity during the day to promote overall health and facilitate better sleep.

7. Limit Caffeine Intake: Avoid giving caffeinated beverages or foods close to bedtime, as caffeine can interfere with sleep.

8. Healthy Bedtime Snack: If hungry before bedtime, offer a light, healthy snack like yogurt or a banana to prevent discomfort without overloading the digestive system.

9. Maintain a Dark Room: Use blackout curtains to create a dark sleeping

environment, promoting the production of melatonin, the sleep-inducing hormone.

10. Comfortable Mattress and Pillows: Ensure the child's mattress and pillows are comfortable and supportive, promoting a restful night's sleep.

11. Open Communication: Encourage open communication about any fears or concerns the child may have that could be impacting their ability to sleep.

12. Limit Sugar Intake: Minimize the intake of sugary foods and drinks, especially close to bedtime, to prevent energy spikes that could disrupt sleep.

13. Avoid Heavy Meals Before Bed: Refrain from serving heavy meals close to bedtime, as they can cause discomfort and indigestion.

14. Create a Relaxing Bedtime Atmosphere: Dim the lights as bedtime approaches to signal that it's time to wind down and prepare for sleep.

15. Consistent Wake-Up Time: Encourage waking up at the same time each day, which helps regulate the child's internal body clock.

16. Encourage Independence: Teach older children to self-soothe and fall asleep independently, promoting healthy sleep habits.

17. Limit Naps: If the child naps during the day, ensure that the naps are age-appropriate and don't interfere with the nightly sleep routine.

18. Promote Positive Associations: Associate bedtime with positive

experiences, such as a favorite bedtime story or a comforting stuffed animal.

19. Regular Eye Check-ups: Ensure the child's eyesight is checked regularly, as vision issues can sometimes contribute to sleep difficulties.

20. Monitor Sleep Quality: Pay attention to signs of sleep disturbances, such as snoring or restlessness, and consult with a healthcare professional if concerns arise.

CHAPTER 4

NAVIGATING THE GROCERY AISLES: A PARENT'S SHOPPING GUIDE

Navigating the grocery aisles as a parent requires strategic planning to ensure a balance between nutritional value, convenience, and the preferences of your family. One practical tip is to create a shopping list before heading to the store. This helps you stay focused, reduces impulse purchases, and ensures you have the necessary ingredients for balanced meals.

Prioritize fresh, whole foods in your shopping list. Vegetables, fruits, lean proteins, and whole grains should form the foundation of your grocery cart. These nutrient-dense items contribute to a well-rounded and healthy diet for your family.

When selecting packaged foods, practice reading nutrition labels. Pay attention to serving sizes, ingredients, and nutritional content. This skill allows you to make informed choices, avoiding products high in added sugars, saturated fats, and unnecessary additives.

Explore different sections of the store to discover healthier alternatives. For example, instead of regular pasta, consider whole-grain or legume-based options. Opt for plain yogurt and add your own fruit to control sugar intake. Small substitutions contribute to a more nutritious overall diet.

Engage your children in the grocery shopping process. Allow them to choose fruits, vegetables, or snacks within predefined healthy options. This involvement not only teaches them about food choices but also makes them more excited about trying new, nutritious foods.

Take advantage of sales and discounts, but be mindful of bulk purchases. While buying in bulk can save money, it's essential to ensure that perishable items won't go to waste before your family can consume them. Consider freezing extras or sharing with neighbors to minimize food waste.

Plan meals for the week ahead, taking into account your family's schedule. This helps streamline your grocery shopping, ensuring you have the necessary ingredients for each meal. It also reduces the likelihood of last-minute, less nutritious choices.

Explore the perimeter of the store first, as this is often where fresh produce, dairy, and proteins are located. These whole foods are essential components of a healthy diet. Once you've covered these areas, venture into the center aisles for specific staples while avoiding overly processed items.

Be mindful of marketing tactics. Products labeled as "natural" or "organic" may still contain unhealthy ingredients. Scrutinize labels and prioritize the nutritional content over marketing claims to make informed choices for your family's well-being.

Consider the environmental impact of your choices. Opt for products with minimal packaging or those that use eco-friendly materials. Choosing locally sourced and seasonal items when possible supports sustainability and community farmers.

Check for unit prices on shelf tags to compare the cost per ounce or pound of different brands and sizes. This helps you make more economical choices, especially when deciding between various packaging options for the same product.

Lastly, don't shop on an empty stomach. Hunger can lead to impulsive and less healthy food choices. Having a balanced meal or snack before shopping ensures you make more rational and nutrition-focused decisions in the grocery aisles.

By incorporating these practical tips into your grocery shopping routine, you can navigate the aisles with confidence, making choices that prioritize your family's health and well-being

Decoding Food Labels for Healthier Choices

Understanding food labels is crucial for making informed and healthier dietary choices. The Nutrition Facts panel provides a wealth of information, starting with serving size. Often, portions differ from what one might consider a typical serving, impacting the accuracy of nutritional intake assessments.

Next, examining the calorie count aids in managing energy consumption. However, not all calories are equal; the source matters. Assessing macronutrients—fats, proteins, and carbohydrates—offers insight into nutritional composition. Optimal ratios vary based on individual needs, emphasizing the importance of personalized dietary approaches.

Delving into the details of fats is essential. While total fat content is highlighted, discerning between saturated, unsaturated, and trans fats is crucial. Prioritizing unsaturated fats, found in sources like avocados and nuts, promotes heart health.

Sodium levels warrant attention, as excessive intake correlates with health issues. Recognizing hidden sources of sodium aids in reducing overall consumption. Similarly, scrutinizing added sugars is imperative. Manufacturers often use various names for sugar, complicating identification. Minimizing added sugars aligns with health-conscious choices.

Fiber is a key player in a balanced diet, influencing digestive health and satiety. Assessing fiber content aids in selecting foods that contribute to overall well-being. Furthermore, understanding protein sources and their quality aids in muscle maintenance and repair.

Decoding ingredient lists unravels the mystery behind processed foods. Prioritizing whole, recognizable ingredients over additives enhances nutritional value. Allergen information is crucial for those with sensitivities, ensuring safe consumption.

Certifications, such as organic or non-GMO, signify specific production practices. Familiarity with these labels empowers consumers to align their choices with personal values. Lastly, expiration dates guide freshness, ensuring food safety.

In essence, decoding food labels involves a comprehensive analysis of serving sizes, calorie content, macronutrient distribution, fats, sodium, sugars, fiber, protein quality, ingredient lists, certifications, and expiration dates. This multifaceted approach empowers individuals to navigate the complexities of food labels, fostering healthier dietary habits.

Smart Snacking Strategies for the Whole Family

Smart snacking is a cornerstone of maintaining a healthy lifestyle for the entire family. Understanding the principles of balanced snacks helps ensure that everyone gets the energy they need without compromising nutritional goals.

Begin by embracing whole foods as the foundation of snacks. Fresh fruits and vegetables make excellent choices, providing essential vitamins, minerals, and fiber. Pairing these with protein-rich options like nut butter or cheese enhances satiety and sustains energy levels.

Nuts and seeds are nutritional powerhouses that offer a blend of healthy fats, protein, and micronutrients. However, portion control is key, as they are calorie-dense. Pre-portioning snacks in small containers helps manage intake and prevents mindless munching.

Yogurt, especially the Greek variety, is an excellent source of protein and probiotics, promoting gut health. Combine it with berries or a drizzle of honey for added flavor and nutritional benefits. Consider incorporating dairy alternatives for those with lactose intolerance.

Whole-grain snacks, such as air-popped popcorn or whole-grain crackers, contribute complex carbohydrates for sustained energy. Paired with hummus or guacamole, they become a satisfying and nutritious option. Avoiding highly processed and refined snacks is crucial for optimizing nutritional value.

Hydration is often overlooked in snacking strategies. Encourage water consumption by infusing it with fruits or herbs for a refreshing twist. Herbal teas or diluted fruit juices can also be alternatives, steering clear of excessive added sugars commonly found in many commercial beverages.

Timing plays a vital role in smart snacking. Be attuned to hunger cues and plan snacks strategically between meals. This prevents overeating during main meals and stabilizes blood sugar levels throughout the day.

Involving the whole family in snack preparation fosters a sense of ownership and encourages healthier choices. Engage children in age-appropriate tasks, such as washing fruits, assembling snack boxes, or even creating simple recipes together.

Mindful snacking involves savoring each bite and paying attention to hunger and fullness cues. Discourage distractions, such as screens, during snack time to promote a mindful eating environment.

Variety is key to preventing snack-time monotony. Rotate through a diverse selection of snacks to expose the family to different flavors and nutrients. This not only keeps things interesting but also ensures a broad spectrum of nutritional benefits.

Consider the nutritional context of the day when planning snacks. If a meal is anticipated within a short timeframe, opt for a lighter snack. Conversely, if there's a longer gap between meals, choose a more substantial option to bridge the hunger gap.

Snacking on the go is inevitable for busy families. Prepare portable snacks like trail mix, pre-cut fruits, or whole-grain bars to avoid relying on less healthy convenience options.

Address specific dietary needs and restrictions within the family when planning snacks. This could involve accommodating allergies, preferences, or cultural considerations to ensure inclusivity.

Maintain an open dialogue about the nutritional value of snacks with the family. Educate them about the benefits of choosing nutrient-dense options and the impact on overall well-being.

Lead by example; when parents prioritize smart snacking, children are more likely to adopt these habits. Demonstrate a positive relationship with food, emphasizing its role in nourishment and enjoyment.

In summary, smart snacking for the whole family involves incorporating a variety of whole foods, embracing portion control, staying hydrated, being mindful, involving the family in preparation, promoting variety, considering timing, and addressing specific dietary needs. By adopting these strategies, families can create a foundation for healthy and enjoyable snacking habits.

CHAPTER 5

MINDFUL PARENTING: CULTIVATING POSITIVE BODY IMAGE

Mindful parenting plays a crucial role in cultivating a positive body image in children. One practical approach is promoting open communication about body image from an early age. Encouraging children to express their feelings and thoughts about their bodies creates a safe space for dialogue, fostering understanding and self-awareness.

Modeling positive behavior is another essential aspect of mindful parenting for positive body image. Parents can demonstrate self-acceptance and speak positively about their own bodies, emphasizing the importance of embracing diversity and rejecting unrealistic beauty standards. Children often emulate the behavior they observe, making parental influence significant in shaping their perceptions.

Encouraging healthy habits without focusing solely on appearance is a practical strategy for mindful parenting. Emphasizing the importance of nutrition and physical activity for overall well-being rather than weight or appearance helps children develop a positive relationship with their bodies. This approach instills a sense of empowerment and self-care.

Promoting media literacy is crucial in mindful parenting to counteract unrealistic body ideals portrayed in the media. Teaching children to critically evaluate media messages and understand that images are often edited or manipulated fosters a more realistic perspective. This awareness helps buffer against negative body image influences.

Creating a body-positive environment at home involves celebrating and respecting different body types. Mindful parents can refrain from making negative comments about their own or others' bodies and instead focus on valuing individuals for their qualities and achievements. This approach reinforces the idea that worth is not determined by appearance.

Emphasizing the importance of self-love and self-compassion is a practical tool in mindful parenting for positive body image. Encouraging children to appreciate their bodies for what they can do rather than how they look fosters a sense of gratitude and acceptance. Teaching self-compassion helps children navigate challenges with resilience.

Addressing bullying and body shaming proactively is essential for mindful parenting. Creating an open dialogue about these issues and teaching children how to respond assertively to negative comments helps build their confidence and resilience. Mindful parents can also collaborate with schools to promote a culture of acceptance and respect.

Encouraging activities that focus on body awareness, such as yoga or mindful movement, is a practical strategy for mindful parenting. These activities help children connect with their bodies in a positive way, fostering a sense of balance and well-being. Incorporating mindfulness practices into daily routines can contribute to a healthier body image.

Setting realistic expectations and avoiding comparisons within the family is important in mindful parenting. Recognizing and celebrating each child's unique qualities and strengths helps prevent unhealthy competition or feelings of inadequacy. This approach fosters an environment where children feel accepted and valued.

Teaching emotional intelligence is a practical tool for mindful parenting in the context of positive body image. Helping children identify and express their emotions, particularly those related to body image, enables them to navigate these feelings in a healthy way. This emotional awareness contributes to a more positive and resilient mindset.

Encouraging a positive relationship with food is crucial for mindful parenting. Avoiding restrictive diets and instead promoting a balanced approach to eating helps children develop a healthy relationship with food and their bodies. Mindful parents can emphasize the importance of enjoying a variety of foods for nourishment and pleasure.

Lastly, fostering a strong sense of self-esteem through praise and encouragement is a practical approach in mindful parenting. Acknowledging children's efforts, accomplishments, and unique qualities helps build their confidence and self-worth. This foundation of self-esteem contributes to a positive body image and resilience in the face of societal pressures.

In summary, mindful parenting for positive body image involves creating an open, supportive, and accepting environment that emphasizes holistic well-being over appearance. By incorporating these practical strategies, parents can help cultivate a healthy body image in their children, setting the stage for a positive relationship with themselves and others.

Fostering a Healthy Relationship with Food.

Maintaining a healthy relationship with food is crucial for overall well-being. It begins with understanding that food is not just fuel for the body but also a source of pleasure and nourishment. Embracing a balanced approach involves appreciating the diverse array of foods available and avoiding restrictive diets that may lead to unhealthy habits.

Mindful eating plays a pivotal role in fostering a healthy relationship with food. Being present during meals, savoring each bite, and paying attention to hunger and fullness cues can help prevent overeating and promote a more intuitive approach to eating. This practice encourages a deeper connection with the sensory experience of food, enhancing enjoyment and satisfaction.

Cultivating a positive mindset towards food involves reframing thoughts and eliminating guilt associated with certain food choices. Rather than labeling foods as "good" or "bad," it's beneficial to view them as part of a broader spectrum that contributes to overall nutritional balance. This mindset shift reduces the likelihood of feeling deprived and promotes a more sustainable, flexible approach to eating.

Creating a supportive environment is essential for nurturing a healthy relationship with food. This involves surrounding oneself with nutritious options at home, making it easier to make positive food choices. Additionally, fostering a sense of community around food, such as cooking and sharing meals with loved ones, can enhance the social aspect of eating and contribute to a positive relationship with food.

Listening to the body's signals is a fundamental aspect of promoting a healthy connection with food. Recognizing true hunger and responding to it with nourishing options allows for a more intuitive and sustainable approach to eating. Likewise, understanding emotional cues that may trigger non-hunger-related eating can help address underlying issues without turning to food as a coping mechanism.

Educating oneself about nutrition is a key component of fostering a healthy relationship with food. Learning about the nutritional value of different foods and understanding individual dietary needs enables informed decision-making, ensuring that meals align with personal health goals. This knowledge empowers individuals to make choices that support their well-being without succumbing to misinformation or trends.

Avoiding extreme or rigid dietary patterns is crucial for promoting a healthy relationship with food. Extreme restrictions and overly prescriptive diets can lead to feelings of deprivation and may contribute to unhealthy eating behaviors. Embracing moderation and flexibility allows for a more sustainable and enjoyable approach to nourishment.

Physical activity complements a healthy relationship with food by contributing to overall well-being. Regular exercise not only supports physical health but also has positive effects on mental and emotional states. Engaging in activities that are enjoyable and align with personal preferences helps create a holistic approach to health that includes both movement and mindful eating.

Understanding the concept of portion control is integral to maintaining a healthy relationship with food. Portion sizes play a significant role in managing calorie intake and promoting balance. Being mindful of appropriate portions contributes to a more realistic and sustainable approach to eating, preventing overconsumption without the need for strict rules.

Meal planning and preparation are practical strategies for fostering a healthy relationship with food. Having nutritious meals readily available reduces reliance on convenient, often less healthy, options. Planning allows for intentional choices, ensuring a well-rounded and varied diet that meets nutritional needs.

Acknowledging and challenging societal pressures and unrealistic body ideals is crucial in developing a positive relationship with food. Focusing on individual health rather than external expectations promotes self-acceptance and reduces the likelihood of engaging in harmful behaviors driven by societal standards.

Celebrating food as a source of pleasure and enjoyment is an essential aspect of fostering a healthy relationship. Allowing oneself to indulge occasionally without guilt contributes to a balanced approach to eating. Finding joy in the culinary experience and appreciating the cultural and social significance of food enhances the overall relationship with nourishment.

Practicing self-compassion is vital for maintaining a healthy relationship with food. Understanding that occasional indulgences or deviations from a routine are a natural part of life helps prevent feelings of failure or guilt. Embracing self-compassion encourages resilience and a positive outlook on the journey towards a healthier lifestyle.

Seeking professional guidance, such as consulting with a registered dietitian or nutritionist, can provide personalized support in developing a healthy relationship with food. These experts can offer tailored advice based on individual needs, preferences, and health goals, helping navigate the vast and sometimes contradictory information surrounding nutrition.

In summary, fostering a healthy relationship with food involves a multifaceted approach encompassing mindfulness, positive mindset, education, and self-compassion. Embracing balance, moderation, and an appreciation for the diverse roles food plays in our lives contributes to long-term well-being and a sustainable, enjoyable approach to nourishment.

Promoting Self-Esteem and Confidence

Promoting self-esteem and confidence is a journey that involves incorporating practical strategies into daily life. One effective approach is acknowledging personal achievements, no matter how small. Celebrating accomplishments, whether completing a task or reaching a goal, fosters a positive self-image and reinforces one's capabilities.

Engaging in positive self-talk is a powerful tool for building self-esteem. Being mindful of inner dialogue and replacing self-critical thoughts with affirming statements helps reshape the way individuals perceive themselves. This practice encourages a more constructive and nurturing relationship with the self.

Setting and accomplishing realistic goals is fundamental to boosting self-esteem. Breaking down larger objectives into manageable steps allows for a sense of accomplishment with each milestone achieved. This gradual progress builds confidence and reinforces the belief that one can overcome challenges.

Cultivating self-care habits contributes significantly to overall well-being and self-esteem. Prioritizing activities that promote physical, mental, and emotional health, such as exercise, adequate sleep, and relaxation, communicates a message of self-worth and fosters a positive self-image.

Developing and maintaining healthy boundaries is crucial for building self-esteem. Clearly expressing personal limits and respecting oneself by saying 'no' when necessary reinforces a sense of autonomy and self-respect. Establishing boundaries promotes healthier relationships and prevents feelings of being overwhelmed.

Surrounding oneself with a supportive and positive social network is essential for boosting self-esteem. Building connections with people who uplift, encourage, and appreciate one's strengths fosters a sense of belonging and reinforces positive self-perception. Healthy relationships provide a foundation for personal growth and confidence.

Practicing gratitude is a simple yet impactful way to enhance self-esteem. Reflecting on and appreciating positive aspects of life, no matter how small, instills a sense of abundance and contentment. This mindset shift contributes to a more optimistic and confident outlook.

Embracing a growth mindset is key to building self-esteem. Viewing challenges as opportunities for learning and growth rather than insurmountable obstacles fosters resilience and a positive attitude towards personal development. A growth mindset encourages a belief in one's ability to improve and adapt.

Engaging in activities that align with personal passions and interests is a powerful way to boost self-esteem. Pursuing hobbies and interests provides a sense of purpose and accomplishment, reinforcing a positive self-image based on individual strengths and talents.

Taking care of physical appearance can positively impact self-esteem. While external factors should not solely define self-worth, grooming and dressing in a way that reflects personal style and comfort can contribute to a positive self-image and increased confidence.

Practicing mindfulness and staying present in the moment is beneficial for building self-esteem. Being aware of thoughts and emotions without judgment allows individuals to respond to challenges with a calm and rational mindset. Mindfulness promotes self-awareness and emotional resilience.

Accepting imperfections and embracing authenticity is crucial for building self-esteem. Recognizing that nobody is perfect and that flaws are a natural part of being human fosters self-compassion. Embracing authenticity allows individuals to feel more comfortable in their own skin, promoting a positive self-image.

Learning from failures and setbacks is a constructive way to build self-esteem. Instead of viewing mistakes as reflections of personal inadequacy, considering them as opportunities for growth and improvement reinforces resilience and a positive self-perception.

Engaging in positive affirmations can be a powerful daily practice for boosting self-esteem. Regularly repeating positive statements about oneself helps reshape subconscious beliefs and reinforces a more positive self-image. Affirmations can be tailored to address specific areas of self-esteem that may need improvement.

Seeking professional support, such as therapy or counseling, can provide valuable tools for building self-esteem. Professionals can help individuals explore underlying issues, develop coping strategies, and provide guidance on building a healthier self-image. Therapy offers a safe space for self-reflection and personal growth.

Promoting self-esteem and confidence involves a combination of self-awareness, positive actions, and a supportive environment. By incorporating these practical strategies into daily life, individuals can cultivate a stronger sense of self-worth, leading to increased confidence and a more fulfilling life.

CHAPTER 6

FAMILY FITNESS: MAKING EXERCISE FUN FOR EVERYONE

Promoting family fitness is key to navigating obesity in kids, fostering a healthy and active lifestyle for the entire family.

Begin by incorporating physical activities that appeal to all age groups. Family-friendly exercises, such as hiking, biking, or even regular walks, can make fitness enjoyable for everyone.

Engage in interactive sports and games. From soccer to family-friendly relay races, these activities not only promote physical health but also strengthen family bonds.

Encourage participation in group fitness classes or home workout sessions. This can be a fun and effective way for family members to exercise together, promoting a sense of unity and shared commitment to health.

Integrate technology in a positive way. Utilize fitness apps or video games that encourage movement, turning exercise into an interactive and enjoyable experience for kids and parents alike.

Plan active outings as a family. Whether it's a day at the beach, a visit to a local park, or exploring nature trails, incorporating physical activities into family outings makes exercise a natural part of the family routine.

Create friendly competitions. Organize family challenges or contests, promoting a sense of friendly rivalry that motivates everyone to stay active and enjoy the benefits of exercise.

Establish a routine that includes physical activity. Designate specific times for family workouts, making it a regular and anticipated part of the day or week.

Involve children in choosing activities. Allowing kids to have a say in the types of exercises or sports the family engages in empowers them and increases their enthusiasm for staying active.

Turn chores into opportunities for movement. Incorporate physical activity into everyday tasks, making chores like gardening, cleaning, or even dancing while tidying up a family affair.

Emphasize the importance of teamwork. Working together towards fitness goals fosters a supportive environment and teaches kids valuable lessons about collaboration and mutual encouragement.

Celebrate milestones and achievements. Acknowledge and reward family members for their dedication to fitness, reinforcing positive behavior and making exercise a positive experience for everyone.

Lead by example. Demonstrate a commitment to a healthy lifestyle through your own actions. When children see their parents prioritizing fitness, they are more likely to adopt similar habits, creating a lasting impact on their overall well-being

Incorporating Playful Activities into Daily Routines

Incorporating playful activities into daily routines is a delightful way to infuse joy, creativity, and a sense of lightheartedness into our lives. Start the morning with a burst of energy by turning the routine of getting dressed into a playful dress-up game. Let children express their creativity by mixing and matching outfits or even experimenting with fun accessories.

Mealtime can become an interactive adventure by incorporating themed dinners or lunches. Choose a theme, and let the family participate in creating decorations, dressing up, or even preparing dishes related to the chosen theme. This not only adds excitement to meals but also encourages collaboration and shared creativity.

Integrate play into daily walks or commutes. Whether it's incorporating a scavenger hunt during a nature walk or playing an audiobook or podcast during the commute, these playful additions make routine activities more enjoyable and mentally engaging.

Transform the mundane task of grocery shopping into a scavenger hunt or a playful learning experience for kids. Create a list of items they need to find, turning the grocery store into a fun exploration while teaching them about different foods and categories.

Utilize technology in a playful manner by engaging in interactive video games that promote physical activity. Platforms like dance or fitness games can turn exercise into a family-friendly competition, making it both entertaining and health-focused.

During work or study breaks, introduce quick brain teasers, riddles, or short mindfulness activities. These playful interludes refresh the mind, enhance focus, and provide a moment of relaxation, contributing to a more productive work or study routine.

Incorporate playful elements into bedtime rituals. Create a bedtime story where each family member contributes a sentence or take turns expressing gratitude for the day. These lighthearted activities create a positive bedtime routine, fostering a sense of connection and warmth.

Create a family challenge or project, such as a DIY art project or a mini-science experiment. This not only brings the family together in a playful setting but also provides an opportunity for shared learning and creative expression.

Turn household chores into a game by setting a timer and challenging family members to complete tasks before it goes off. This adds an element of competition, making chores more enjoyable and turning them into a group effort.

Embrace spontaneous dance parties or "movement moments" throughout the day. Play a favorite song and encourage everyone to join in for a quick dance break, infusing the routine with energy and laughter.

Explore outdoor activities as a family, whether it's playing sports, going for a bike ride, or having a picnic. Outdoor play not only promotes physical well-being but also allows for a change of scenery, making daily routines more dynamic and enjoyable.

Cap off the day with a family game night, featuring board games, card games, or even video games that encourage friendly competition and laughter. This dedicated time for play fosters strong family bonds and provides a joyful conclusion to the day.

Creating a Supportive and Active Family Culture to navigate obesity in kids

Creating a supportive and active family culture is instrumental in navigating obesity in kids, fostering a lifestyle that prioritizes health and well-being for the entire family.

Begin by establishing open communication about health and nutrition. Engage in discussions about the importance of a balanced diet, the benefits of physical activity, and the potential consequences of a sedentary lifestyle. Creating a dialogue around these topics helps build awareness and understanding within the family.

Lead by example. Demonstrate a commitment to an active lifestyle by engaging in regular exercise and making nutritious food choices. Children are more likely to adopt healthy habits when they see their parents actively participating in them, creating a positive family culture around well-being.

Make physical activity a family affair. Plan and participate in activities that everyone can enjoy, such as family walks, bike rides, or sports. This not only promotes bonding but also ensures that everyone in the family is actively involved in maintaining a healthy lifestyle.

Incorporate fitness into family outings. Choose recreational activities that involve movement, such as visiting parks, going on nature hikes, or spending a day at the beach. This transforms outings into opportunities for both fun and physical activity.

Establish consistent mealtime routines. Eating together as a family fosters a sense of connection and allows for positive role modeling of healthy eating habits. Create an environment where meals are seen as enjoyable, shared experiences rather than just a necessity.

Encourage extracurricular activities that involve physical movement. Whether it's organized sports, dance classes, or outdoor adventures, supporting and participating in these activities helps instill a love for movement in children and reinforces an active family culture.

Limit screen time and promote alternatives. Establish guidelines for recreational screen time and encourage alternative activities that involve physical movement, such as playing outside, engaging in creative projects, or participating in family-friendly fitness challenges.

Involve children in meal planning and preparation. This not only educates them about nutrition but also gives them a sense of ownership over their food choices. Create a positive and collaborative atmosphere in the kitchen, making healthy eating a family effort.

Celebrate achievements together. Acknowledge and celebrate milestones related to physical activity and healthy habits. This positive reinforcement strengthens the family's commitment to an active lifestyle and motivates everyone to continue making health-conscious choices.

Create a supportive environment for emotional well-being. Address stressors and challenges as a family, emphasizing the importance of mental health. Engage in activities that promote relaxation and bonding, such as family game nights or mindfulness exercises.

Establish regular health check-ups for everyone in the family. Monitoring physical health, growth, and development ensures early detection and intervention if any health concerns arise. This proactive approach contributes to a supportive family culture centered around well-being.

Encourage a positive body image. Foster an environment where everyone feels accepted and valued regardless of their body size. Emphasize the importance of overall health and well-being rather than focusing solely on appearance, promoting a healthy relationship with one's body.

CHAPTER 7

SUSTAINING CHANGE: LONG-TERM HABITS FOR LIFELONG WELLNESS

Sustaining change in children's habits is crucial for lifelong wellness, especially in combating obesity. It requires a holistic approach encompassing nutrition, physical activity, and mental well-being.

Parents play a pivotal role in fostering long-term habits. Inculcate healthy eating patterns by involving children in meal planning and grocery shopping, making them aware of nutritious choices.

Ensure a balanced diet with a variety of fruits, vegetables, whole grains, and lean proteins. Educate children about the benefits of each food group, promoting an understanding of nutritional values.

Incorporate enjoyable physical activities into daily routines. This can be achieved through sports, outdoor play, or family activities, promoting a positive association with exercise.

Set limits on screen time to encourage physical activity and reduce sedentary behavior. Promote alternative activities like reading, playing board games, or engaging in creative pursuits.

Foster healthy snacking habits by having a selection of nutritious snacks readily available. Replace sugary snacks with options like fruits, nuts, or yogurt.

Instill the habit of drinking water regularly. Limit sugary beverages and educate children on the importance of staying hydrated for overall health.

Establish a consistent sleep routine. Ensure that children get adequate sleep as it plays a vital role in metabolism and overall well-being.

Reinforce positive behaviors with non-food rewards. Encourage and praise healthy choices, fostering a sense of accomplishment.

Educate children about the impact of food choices on their health. This knowledge empowers them to make informed decisions about their diet.

Create a supportive family environment where everyone participates in adopting healthy habits. This collective effort reinforces the importance of wellness.

Conduct regular check-ins to assess progress and address challenges. Open communication allows for adjustments in the approach to better suit the child's needs, ensuring sustained change in the long run.

Celebrating Milestones and Embracing a Healthy Future

Celebrating milestones and embracing a healthy future is integral in Overcoming obesity in kids. Acknowledging and rewarding achievements contributes to the child's motivation and creates positive associations with a healthier lifestyle.

When milestones are reached, whether they involve dietary improvements or increased physical activity, take the time to celebrate. This can be done through verbal praise, small non-food rewards, or engaging in a special activity the child enjoys.

Encourage the child to actively participate in setting and tracking their goals. This involvement fosters a sense of ownership and responsibility, making them more likely to stay committed to healthier habits.

Celebrate not only weight-related achievements but also behavioral changes. Recognize improved self-esteem, increased energy levels, and enhanced overall well-being, emphasizing the holistic benefits of a healthier lifestyle.

Involve the entire family in celebrations. This collective recognition reinforces a supportive environment and highlights that health and well-being are shared family goals.

Create a visual representation of milestones achieved. This could be a chart, a journal, or a simple record that allows the child to see their progress and reflect on how far they've come.

Use celebrations as opportunities for education. Discuss the positive impacts of healthier choices on the child's body and emphasize the long-term benefits of maintaining these habits.

Introduce new and exciting activities as rewards. This could involve a family outing, a day of exploring nature, or trying out a new sport. The aim is to associate positive experiences with a healthier lifestyle.

Emphasize the importance of balance in celebrations. While it's crucial to recognize achievements, it's equally important not to undermine progress by indulging excessively in unhealthy behaviors.

Encourage the child to share their achievements with peers or friends. Positive social reinforcement can further motivate them to continue making healthy choices.

As the child progresses, revisit and adjust goals to reflect new challenges and aspirations. This adaptability ensures that the journey toward a healthier future remains engaging and relevant.

In the conclusion, remember that celebrating milestones and embracing a healthy future is a continuous process. It's not just about reaching a specific weight but instilling lifelong habits that contribute to overall well-being.

In navigating obesity in kids, the focus should be on cultivating a positive relationship with food, fostering a love for physical activity, and nurturing mental well-being. By celebrating milestones, both big and small, we contribute to shaping a healthy and fulfilling future for our children.

CONCLUSION

In conclusion, "Healthy Habits, Happy Kids: Navigating the Challenges of Childhood Obesity" emphasizes the significance of cultivating positive habits early on to promote the well-being of our children. The journey outlined in this book underscores that addressing childhood obesity requires a multifaceted approach that encompasses nutrition, physical activity, and mental health.

Throughout these pages, we've delved into practical strategies for building and sustaining healthy habits. From balanced nutrition and regular physical activity to fostering a positive body image and supporting mental well-being, every aspect contributes to a child's overall health and happiness.

The importance of parental involvement has been a consistent theme, recognizing that caregivers play a pivotal role in shaping a child's habits. By setting realistic goals, celebrating milestones, and creating a supportive family environment, we empower both parents and children to navigate the challenges of childhood obesity together.

The journey toward a healthier lifestyle is not without its obstacles, and this book acknowledges the realities of the modern world. From the temptations of processed foods to the allure of screens, we've explored practical ways to overcome these challenges and instill habits that last a lifetime.

Education has been a cornerstone of our approach, emphasizing the need to equip children with the knowledge to make informed choices about their health. By fostering an understanding of nutrition, the benefits of exercise, and the importance of mental well-being, we empower our children to take an active role in their own health journey.

As we conclude, it's essential to recognize that the path to a healthier future is ongoing. Healthy habits are not a destination but a lifelong journey. By embracing this reality, we lay the foundation for a generation of children who not only overcome the challenges of obesity but also thrive in a life filled with vitality and happiness.

"Healthy Habits, Happy Kids" is not just a book; it's a guide for parents, caregivers, and educators dedicated to shaping a brighter and healthier future for our children.

May the insights shared within these pages inspire positive changes and contribute to a world where every child has the opportunity to grow up healthy, happy, and full of potential.

Please, **click on** the link below to connect and check more excellent books

https://amazon.com/author/juliantim4kids